The Ul Guide To Menopause

Wisdom And Diet Every Women Should Know To Get Through Menopause Easily

Elizabeth Grace

Table of Contents

Introduction

Chapter 1: Understanding Menopause

Chapter 2: Hormones are the Root of it All

Chapter 3: Signs of Times

Chapter 4: Facing Menopause Head-On

Chapter 5: What You Eat Matters

Chapter 6: What is the Wisdom Behind Menopause?

Conclusion

Introduction

I want to thank you and congratulate you for purchasing the book, *"The Ultimate guide To Menopause: Wisdom And Diet Every Women Should Know To Get Through Menopause Easily"*.

This book contains proven steps and strategies on how to get through the menopausal stage by understanding what it is all about.

This book is written for every woman out there. Whether you are approaching menopause, going through it or past it, this book is about you and the challenges of the menopausal stage that you will encounter or that you might have already overcome.

I hope this book gives you the knowledge you need to face this next chapter of your life. I hope it gives you courage. I hope it empowers you to claim and enjoy your life as a woman, no matter what stage in your life you might find yourself in.

Thanks again for purchasing this book, I hope you enjoy it!

© **Copyright 2014 by Elizabeth Grace - All rights reserved.**

This document is geared towards providing exact and reliable information in regards to the topic and issue covered. The publication is sold with the idea that the publisher is not required to render accounting, officially permitted, or otherwise, qualified services. If advice is necessary, legal or professional, a practiced individual in the profession should be ordered.

- From a Declaration of Principles which was accepted and approved equally by a Committee of the American Bar Association and a Committee of Publishers and Associations.

In no way is it legal to reproduce, duplicate, or transmit any part of this document in either electronic means or in printed format. Recording of this publication is strictly prohibited and any storage of this document is not allowed unless with written permission from the publisher. All rights reserved.

The information provided herein is stated to be truthful and consistent, in that any liability, in terms of inattention or otherwise, by any usage or abuse of any policies, processes, or directions contained within is the solitary and utter responsibility of the recipient reader. Under no circumstances will any legal responsibility or blame be held against the publisher for any reparation, damages, or monetary loss due to the information herein, either directly or indirectly.

Respective authors own all copyrights not held by the publisher.

The information herein is offered for informational purposes solely, and is universal as so. The presentation of the information is without contract or any type of guarantee assurance.

The trademarks that are used are without any consent, and the publication of the trademark is without permission or backing by the trademark owner. All trademarks and brands within this book are for clarifying purposes only and are the owned by the owners themselves, not affiliated with this document.

Chapter 1: Understanding Menopause

Menopause—a word feared by many women.

Over time, the word menopause became associated with a lot of negativity. Some may look at it as the beginning of the end as it often signifies the end of a woman's child bearing years. It is not uncommon for some women to feel a sense of worthlessness in knowing that their ability to reproduce is over. Some may feel a sense of loss. Others look at it as a phase in life that is full of hot flashes, bone loss, and just an overall decline in health. It is a dreary and very unappealing life to look forward to.

Many women go through their menopause years clueless on what will happen, how it will happen, and how long it will last. They just woke up one day feeling that something is not right with their bodies. Because of these, they often find themselves scared, confused, and apprehensive. They have no idea what is happening to them. They feel lost and alone, thinking that something is wrong with their bodies.

Understanding what menopause is all about will help appease these fears. It is not a disease or condition that needs to be cured. It is a natural stage in life that every woman will go through. No one can control it. It is something that is inevitable. Knowing why it happens and how it happens will help women deal with this new stage in their lives in the most effective way possible. It will show them how they can continue to enjoy their prime years while managing the symptoms and signs of reaching menopause.

Menopause is not the end. It is in fact the beginning of a new phase in their lives. Knowledge and understanding will liberate them and give them the freedom to enjoy the next chapter in their lives.

To understand menopause, it is important to start with the basics.

The word menopause itself literally means the "end of the cycles" from the root word *men* (month) and the Greek word *pausis* which means cessation. The word describes a stage in a woman's life when menstruation stops permanently, thus marking the end of her ability to reproduce.

Menopause is the opposite of menarche. Menarche defines the stage in a young woman's life when menstruation begins. Her ovaries start producing eggs. At this point in her life, she becomes capable of bearing children.

During menopause, a woman's ovaries are considered officially out of business. They will cease operations and become inactive. It is scientifically defined as the absence of menstrual flow or periods and this will happen once the ovaries themselves have stopped their primary functions.

The ovaries are the core parts of a woman's reproductive system. She has two of these almond-shaped glands. Each month, an ovary produces an egg or ovum. These ovaries are also responsible for producing hormones which in turn, causes the walls of the uterus to thicken, ideally preparing it for implantation of a fertilized egg. If fertilization does not happen, the uterus will later on shed or discard the uterine lining. These are the menses or period that a woman experiences each month. When menopause occurs, all of these activities inside a woman's body will stop permanently.

The common misconception of menopause is that it happens at a certain age or year in woman's life. This is not necessarily the case.

It is a natural phase in a woman's life and just like any phase in life, it is also made up of several stages. The transition from the reproductive state to being non-reproductive is a gradual process. It is not something that happens over night. It occurs over a certain number of years. It starts around late 40s or early 50s and may go on for a few more years or even a decade.

There are four stages of menopause that a woman will go through. Knowing when they will happen will help women brace themselves in facing the years leading up to menopause and the years after that:

Premenopause

This is the term used to describe the years leading up to the last menstruation. This happens around mid to late 40s. There might be no glaring symptoms yet but at this point, the levels of reproductive hormones are beginning to wane.

Perimenopause

This term refers to the transition years to menopause. The events that happen and the changes that occur in their bodies during these years are often incorrectly associated with the term menopause.

The word's literal meaning is "around menopause." This is often considered as the dreaded stage. The North American Menopause Society estimates that this stage can last for four to eight years while The Centre for Menstrual Cycle and Ovulation Research said that it can last up to ten years!

At this point, hormone levels become erratic. There are high points, like estrogen levels reaching by more than 20% to 30%, and there are also low points when hormones levels drop significantly. These fluctuations will often manifest physically. This is when a woman begins to experience the infamous symptoms of what they often thought of as "menopause." The more accurate term to use is actually the perimenopause phase.

Some of these symptoms are hot flashes, vaginal dryness, mood swings, sweating, palpitations, decreased libido, osteoporosis or bone loss, and trouble sleeping (These symptoms and their management will be tackled in detail in the later chapters.).

Though some may feel the signs of the transition phase as early as age 35, most symptoms become evident once a woman hits her late 40s. And since this stage can last up to ten years, a woman's body will go through a lot of changes as her body continues to adjust to the constant up and down of hormones.

Menopause

This stage is clinically defined as the date exactly twelve months after a woman last had her menstrual flow. At this point, the ovaries have officially ceased their functions. They have stopped producing eggs and most of the estrogen in the body.

Postmenopause

This stage pretty much comprises the years ahead, after one year of no menstrual period at all or menopause. As the level of reproductive hormones continues to drop (until the ovaries become inactive), the occurrences of the dreaded symptoms also start to go away. Any spotting or bleeding that may occur during these years is not normal and should be brought to a doctor's attention right away.

Chapter 2: Hormones are the Root of it All

Hormones play a big part during menopause. They explain a lot why women experience a lot of changes in their bodies during menopause. They are the reasons behind those often awful symptoms and discomforts women go through during the perimenopause stage. Understanding what they are and how they work will give women a better understanding of the changes that are happening inside their bodies.

Hormones are defined as chemicals that are naturally secreted by various glands in a human body. These chemical secretions travel all over the blood stream from one body organ to another. They are considered the body's messengers as they communicate with the different parts of the body and affect the different processes in the body like growth, metabolism, reproduction and even moods and emotions. Too little or too much of these hormones are always not a good thing and may cause unwanted changes in the body.

The ovaries are the focus glands in this chapter. This is because they are the glands responsible for producing the hormones that play crucial roles during menopause.

Ovaries are a tiny pair of glands shaped like almonds and are located on opposite sides of the uterus, in the female pelvic cavity. They produce the female sex hormones estrogen and progesterone and all throughout the years after menarche up until puberty, a woman will experience an ebb and flow of these hormones. Estrogen is considered the more dominant hormone.

Estrogen and Progesterone

During puberty, estrogen is the hormone liable for the development of a woman's mammary glands or breasts tissues and her uterus. During the menstrual cycle, this hormone develops the uterine lining. During the menstrual cycle, as the estrogen surges, the menses stop, the uterine lining thickens, and the follicles in the ovary begin to develop, from which an ovum or egg is eventually released in a process called ovulation. Progesterone, on the other hand, which is produced upon ovulation, prepares the uterus for the likelihood of pregnancy as well as the mammary glands for possible lactation. Together, these two hormones work hand in hand during the menstrual cycle. If the egg is not fertilized and no implantation occurs after about two weeks, the levels of these hormones drop and cause the uterus to shed its unused lining. The shedding process is the monthly period that a woman experiences each month.

While these two hormones are commonly associated with the reproductive system, it is important to know that they also play crucial roles in other parts of the body. Estrogen for example is also responsible for calcium absorption which leads to stronger bones. It also plays a role in a woman's bladder and urethral health.

The body is working continuously to balance these hormones but certain factors, both internal and external, can cause changes in the levels of these hormones. When this happens, the body will try to cope with the changes and this is often manifested by various physical symptoms. Some factors that can alter the balance of hormones in the body are stress, medication, and change in body weight, pregnancy and menopause. Though majority of these factors are temporary in nature, menopause on the other hand, is not. It brings about permanent change in the body's hormone levels. When a woman reaches the menopause phase, her ovaries will stop producing eggs. And when that happens, they will also shut off production of estrogen and progesterone.

When a woman reaches her late 30s, her body starts to produce less progesterone. This is made apparent by heavier flows during periods. However, most of the physical signs and symptoms will show when the body's production of estrogen starts to diminish. It is at this point that the body experiences the discomforts that are often associated with the perimenopause phase.

Chapter 3: Signs of Times

As the body's production of vital female hormones such as estrogen comes to a halt during menopause, a woman will start to experience a wide array of physical and emotional symptoms caused by hormonal imbalance. It may seem overwhelming and disheartening to know that this hormonal rollercoaster of highs and lows (or fluctuations) will happen for a couple of years or even more. However, knowing what they are and understanding why they are happening will help alleviate some of these negative feelings. It will also help when considering options in managing these symptoms.

Below are the three most common signs of menopause:

Hot Flashes

Hot flashes are the most popular symptoms among women. Oftentimes, when asked what menopause is, people will often think of hot flashes. What are hot flashes exactly and why are they called such?

A sudden temporary spike in the body temperature due to hormone fluctuations is responsible for hot flashes. When this happens, the body's external temperature surges rapidly and then slowly goes back to normal. These flashes are often accompanied by flushing, sweating and at times, light headedness. Duration and frequency varies and can happen anytime of the day. When they happen at night, they are often called night sweats.

How do you know that you are experiencing hot flashes? If you answered "yes" to most of the questions below, chances are you are having hot flashes:

- Do you experience a sudden intense feeling of heat emanating from all parts of your body especially on the neck, arms and torso?

- Do you notice your face reddening or flushing?

- Do you feel your heart suddenly palpitating?

- Does your pulse quicken?

- Do you experience perspiration and chills?

- Do you suffer from dizziness, nausea, and, at times, headaches?

Vaginal Dryness

Many women are embarrassed about it but this is a normal occurrence during the transition years to menopause. It was revealed in studies that about 40% to 60% of women experience vaginal dryness during the perimenopause stage. This is primarily due to the continuously dwindling levels of estrogen in a woman's body.

The blood vessels in a woman's vaginal wall secrete a clear fluid providing natural lubrication. Vaginal dryness or atrophic vaginitis happens when there is lack of adequate moisture in the vaginal area.

Go over the questions below and find out if you are experiencing vaginal dryness:

- Do you suffer from itching?

- Has intercourse been painful lately? And do you experience light bleeding after?

- Do you experience a burning and stinging sensation down there?

- Do you feel an unexplained pressure on your vaginal area?

- Do you feel discomfort when wearing tight pants?

- Are you urinating more frequently than usual?

- Do you experience general discomfort in the vaginal area?

Mood Swings

The seemingly unending fluctuations of hormones also have a tremendous effect on a woman's emotions and moods. And just like her hormone levels, her moods also go through peaks and lows, oftentimes abrupt and extreme. It is like a pendulum that swings rapidly almost to the point of going out of control.

Estrogen influences the production of serotonin which is commonly known as the mood chemical. It is a chemical produced by the body that acts as a neurotransmitter. It is popularly known to affect and balance a person's moods and emotions. Other symptoms of transition to menopause like night sweats, fatigue and hot flashes can also cause irritability and mood swings. These triggers however, are still caused by hormonal imbalance.

Below are some questions you can go through to assess if you are experiencing mood swings:

- Do you feel an unexplainable surge of emotions like sadness, anger, and depression?

- Do you find yourself lacking the drive or motivation to go through the day?

- Have you been impatient, aggressive and irritable lately towards things that you normally don't pay much attention to?

- Are you feeling more and more stressed lately?

- Do you experience bouts of anxiety and nervousness and doesn't know why?

- Have you been feeling more and more melancholic lately?

No Sex Drive

Probably the most discomforting, sensitive, and embarrassing symptom of perimenopause for most women is the loss of libido. Many women are not comfortable talking about it because they don't want to be deemed inadequate. Not only have they lost the ability to reproduce, they now also find themselves unable to satisfy their partner's sexual desires. This, however, is normal and many women going through menopause experience this.

During this time, many women lose interest in engaging in sexual activities. They may find themselves having less and less sexual feelings toward their partners. Other factors that may contribute to low or no sex drive are vaginal dryness and irritation, as well as mood swings. Again, these are all due to the dwindling presence of female sex hormones in a woman's body.

Below are some questions you can go through to find if you are losing your libido:

- Have you been feeling less and less attracted, sexually, to your partner?

- Do you find yourself becoming less responsive to things that used to stimulate you sexually?

- Do you often think of sex now as more of a chore than an activity that you enjoy?

- Do you lack energy for sex?

The four highlighted symptoms are the most common among many women. The list of symptoms however, is much longer. Here are some of them. Do take note that the symptoms are not limited to those that are listed below:

- Hair loss

- Fatigue

- Memory lapses

- Bloating

- Digestive problems

- Bone loss or osteoporosis

- Incontinence or other urinary health issues

- Weight gain

- Sleep disorders like insomnia

- Irregular periods

Knowing the pains and discomfort that come with the perimenopause years will equip women, especially the younger ones, with knowledge on how to deal with these issues when the time comes. As early as their 30s, women can start looking into possible lifestyle changes to diminish the symptoms that hormonal imbalance will bring upon their bodies.

Chapter 4: Facing Menopause Head-On

Now that you are aware of the mechanisms behind menopause, its different stages, and its long list of symptoms, the next step is for you to decide how you will manage these symptoms for you to be able to continue to enjoy life until your prime years. You should not be a slave to the pains and discomforts of your perimenopause phase. You don't have to wait it out until the symptoms go away. You can take charge of your body and use the knowledge that you have about menopause, to create a course of action that will most suit your body and your lifestyle.

There are five ways to manage perimenopause symptoms. The first option is to go the hormonal route. The second is choosing nonhormonal medication. The third option is the natural way. The third option has three choices under it.

Going Hormonal

Hormone Replacement Therapy or HRT is a popular and controversial way to manage the symptoms of menopause. The therapy's ultimate purpose is to replace the hormones that are no longer produced by a woman's body namely, estrogen and progesterone. There are two types of HRT. The first one is Estrogen Replacement Therapy and the second one is a combination of both hormones.

There are many ways to get these replacement hormones inside a woman's body. The most common is the estrogen pill. It is the top choice because it is convenient, inexpensive and very easy to administer. Estrogen can also be administered by using a patch. This is best for women who have the tendency to forget taking their estrogen pills on a daily basis. The patch is only applied about once or twice a week. Patches though may fall off especially during rigorous activities. Estrogen can also come in forms of creams or gels. They are often applied once or twice daily. These are however not regulated by FDA therefore, were not tested for safety. Estrogen can also be delivered via a hypodermic needle. Injections however are not widely used in the US. They are not convenient and usually require a visit to the doctor to administer the hormones. There are also estrogen vaginal creams available which are often used to manage vaginal dryness. Some hormones are also administered by inserting estrogen pellets under the skin. This process is not too popular as this also requires a visit to the doctor.

Nonhormonal

There are also medications available that can combat and alleviate menopausal symptoms. Many can be taken orally and they don't alter the body's hormone levels.

Some antidepressants were found to be effective in elevating the body's serotonin which helps treat hot flashes and mood swings. Examples of these antidepressant medications are paroxetine, fluoxetine, and venlafaxine. Nonetheless, as much as these medications are effective, they also have side effects like dry mouth, constipation, nausea, insomnia and headaches.

Anti-seizure medication like Gabapentin is also used to reduce hot flashes.

High blood pressure medication clonidine is also another popular nonhormonal medication that helps reduce hot flashes. It has the same effects as the antidepressants sans the mood enhancement part.

There are also vitamin supplements that can be taken to help alleviate the frequency of hot flashes. These are Magnesium and Vitamins E and B.

Going All Natural

Though some women may consider using hormones or medication effective in combating the symptoms of the perimenopause stage, there are those who chose to counteract the effects of hormonal imbalance the natural way.

Oriental Medicine

Alternative medicine like acupuncture is believed to ease hot flashes and other menopausal discomforts. Developed in Asia, this treatment uses very thin needles to activate the flow of vital life force energy in the body. The needles are inserted under the skin to relieve pain and enhance the body's well-being.

Acupressure is another practice that is also gaining popularity. Instead of needles, this technique uses finger point pressure. The pressure points, when activated are believed to release tension, ease pain and enhance the circulation of oxygen and nutrients in the body.

Herbs

Use of herbal remedies is also gaining popularity among women who wish to manage their menopausal symptoms the natural way. Some examples of these are licorice and ginseng. Others include red clover and black cohosh (a plant native to North America). The downside of using herbal remedies is that they are often not regulated by the FDA and some may contain toxins that might bring more harm to the body. For example, further studies of the effect of black cohosh showed that it can cause high liver toxicity. Therefore, it is best to consult first with a trained herbalist or a doctor before dabbing into these herbal remedies.

Yoga and Meditation

Meditation is a practice that has been used for hundreds of years to calm the body, mind, and spirit. When meditating, a person trains the mind to focus the energy on certain body parts to receive healing. It helps lower the blood pressure and regulate breathing and heartbeat. It can also help improve the immune system. Meditation also trains the mind to rid itself of negative thoughts thus alleviating depression which can also be brought about by hormonal imbalance.

Yoga is another practice that can provide physical, mental, and emotional benefits to women going through the perimenopausal phase. It is an ancient discipline that aims to transform and unite the body, mind and spirit through meditation and the practice of different poses or asanas. During the practice of yoga the body is trained to hold poses while focusing on the breath. This in turn helps calm the body including one's heartbeat and pulse. The poses can also include some hip openers and stretches that can help strengthen the vaginal wall and pelvis. There are also poses that help maintain core strength and joint and muscle flexibility, making the body more limber and less prone to injuries.

Lifestyle Changes

As a person ages, the body also ages. There will come a point when a change in lifestyle will become necessary not because the person is feeling his or her age but simply because the body can no longer take all the partying and sleepless nights.

Maintaining a healthy lifestyle can be beneficial in the long run especially for women. Once they hit the menopausal stage, they will reap the fruits of the lifestyle choices they made when they were younger.

Here some lifestyle changes that can help women during their menopausal phase:

- Kick the habit. If you're smoking, now is the time to give it up. Smoking has bad effects not just on the lungs but also on the bones, heart, and blood pressure too.

- Watch the weight. You don't have to be skinny. You just need to keep a healthy body weight, one that is fit for your age.

- Keep it cool. Keep your room cool. Choose clothes that are airy and those that don't trap heat. If the temperature is cold where you are at, dress in layers so that it will be easier for you to remove them when hot flashes occur.

- Relax. Lessen your stress level as much and as often as you can.

- Laugh and smile more. Maintain a positive outlook as much as you can.

- Maintain a healthy relationship with your friends and families. They will be your best support group when times get rough.

Given the numerous options available to battle the discomforts that come with the menopausal stage, it would be very tempting to select the easiest and most convenient way. Keep in mind though that in the end, your decision will depend on what your body tells you it needs. Seek out the help of professionals. Know all your options but be very critical about them. Know all the pros and the cons. Write down what works for you and what doesn't. Research and ask questions. Weigh them carefully. And finally, listen to your body.

Chapter 5: What You Eat Matters

Nutrition during the menopausal years plays a crucial role in combating the discomfort and symptoms that come with it. Your body uses whatever you feed it when adapting to the changes that is happening inside it. If you are feeding it poorly, then, chances are, you are not doing yourself any favor. Your body needs all the support it can get and good nutrition is one of them.

Go Easy On...

Fats. Cut down on saturated fats. Say goodbye to French fries, ice cream and full cream milk. Lessen your intake of trans fats which are often found in baked goods (yes, those cakes and yummy desserts). They increase the risk of heart disease and high blood pressure.

Salt and Sugar. Use them in moderation. Too much sugar can increase the likelihood of diabetes. Sugar is also a culprit for weight gains. Too much sodium on the other hand has been linked to high blood pressure as well as some urinary health problems.

Alcohol. Limit the margaritas and mojitos. A glass or two is enough. Binge drinking days are over. Too much alcohol can hasten bone loss. Plus, not to mention the damages it can cause to your liver.

Fizzy drinks. Yes, soda and other carbonated drinks can hamper calcium absorption. Eating all those dairy products and calcium-rich foods will go to waste if your body can't absorb them.

Spicy foods. These can make those hot flashes soar through the roof.

Coffee and tea. These are stimulants that can also add body heat and worsen hot flashes. They are also known to hinder body absorption of nutrients.

Focus More On...

Calcium. Keep your bones strong and healthy. Drink and eat two to four servings of dairy and food rich in calcium daily. Examples of food rich in calcium are sardines, salmon, broccoli and legumes. Calcium supplements are also available.

Iron. Eat about three servings of food rich in iron like red meat, green leafy vegetables, fish and poultry. Iron helps maintain a healthy immune system.

Fiber. Load up on fiber by eating foods like whole-grain breads, cereals, brown rice, pasta, fruits and vegetables. Fiber cleanses your body and helps it get rid of toxins.

During menopausal stage, it is important to maintain a balanced diet. Too much of anything is bad. Always keep your food intake in moderation. Read the labels of the food that you eat. Know what you are eating. Every time you eat, think of your body and how the food that you ingested will affect it. With this in mind, you will be more watchful of the food that you eat. Your body is your only ally so you have to be mindful of every food that it takes in. You are the only person responsible for its health and well-being.

Chapter 6: What is the Wisdom Behind Menopause?

It was defined in earlier chapters that menopause means the end of a woman's fertility. This concept might seem overwhelming and devastating. Well, that is one way to look at it. But, as the cliché goes, there are always two ways that you can look at things—either your glass is half full or half empty. Menopause might signify the end of your childbearing yours but, it can also mean new beginnings.

Dr. Christiane Northrup—women's health expert, speaker and author of the book *The Wisdom of Menopause* (wherein she debunks many myths about midlife)—calls menopause the "renaissance of a woman's life." And no one could have said it better. She is correct. It is a rebirth. A woman's life does not end because she stopped bearing children. She is just closing a chapter in her life and opening a new one.

Consider the next chapter of your life, the post menopause years, a blank slate. Take it as an opportunity to learn new things that can enrich your life and relationships. When something is taken away, it creates space for something new and better to come. It can be a new career, a new knowledge, a new outlook in life, anything! The possibilities are just endless.

Reaching the menopausal stage in life can shake up a lot of your beliefs and assumptions in life. You will learn to redefine yourself and be open to new things, new thinking and new ideals. You are more than a mother and a wife. Your definition is not limited to the fact that you can bear children. They go beyond that. Thus, some women find themselves at a loss when menopause sets in. Maybe because at some point in their lives, they have confined themselves to being just mothers and wives. And now that they have reached the end of their child bearing years, they are confronted with the challenge of changing the way they perceive themselves. They don't stop being mothers and wives simply because they have grown old and can no longer bear children. Their roles will continue no matter what changes their bodies will go through.

In the end, it is all about finding peace and balance between the unavoidable changes happening in your body and finding a way to ride through them, the best way you can. You accept what you can't change and then you study and try to understand it. After that, you use your knowledge and understanding to allow yourself to adapt to the changes. You adjust your ideals, your beliefs and even your body to the changes. You become flexible in all aspects of your life. And then, you move forward and you carry on.

Acknowledging that your body is forever changing will liberate you from fidgeting over things that you cannot control. Menopause is one of the things in your life you won't be able to stop from happening. It is not a disease or condition that needs treatment. It is a part of life. Every woman will go through it. It is just a matter time. You don't fight against nature. You embrace it and work through it. Understanding what it is and how it happens will help you accept the inevitable. Don't mistake this for surrender. Acceptance is different in a sense that you don't acknowledge defeat. What you acknowledge is the fact that it is part of life and so you find a way to work through it, hopeful that you will survive it and come out a better person – mentally, physically, emotionally, and spiritually.

Conclusion

Thank you again for purchasing this book!

I hope this book was able to help you to understand what menopause is all about.

The next step is to share everything that you have learned in this book to your friends, loved ones, and to all the women out there. Give them the gift of knowledge and empowerment. Share this book to them.

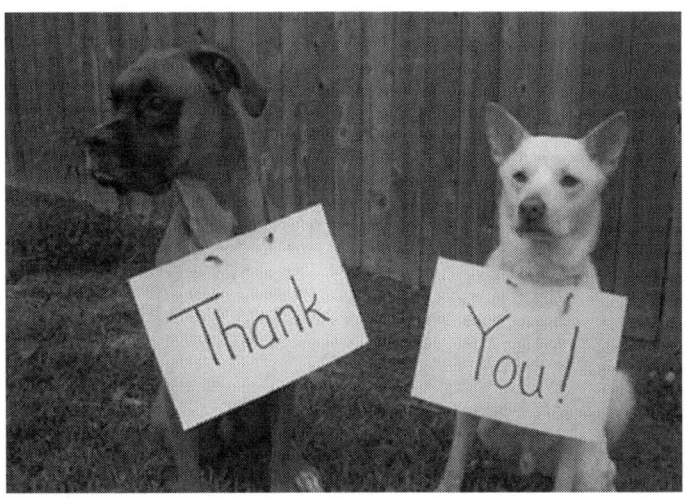

Finally, if you enjoyed this book, then I'd like to ask you for a favor, would you be kind enough to leave a review for this book on Amazon? It'd be greatly appreciated!

Thank you and good luck!

Printed in Poland
by Amazon Fulfillment
Poland Sp. z o.o., Wrocław